70 Of The Best Ever Scrumptious Vegan Dinner Recipes....Revealed!

Samantha Michaels

KU-351-161

Table of Contents

Samantha Michaels

Publishers Notes

Disclaimer

This publication is intended to provide helpful and informative material. It is not intended to diagnose, treat, cure, or prevent any health problem or condition, nor is intended to replace the advice of a physician. No action should be taken solely on the contents of this book. Always consult your physician or qualified health-care professional on any matters regarding your health and before adopting any suggestions in this book or drawing inferences from it.

The author and publisher specifically disclaim all responsibility for any liability, loss or risk, personal or otherwise, which is incurred as a consequence, directly or indirectly, from the use or application of any contents of this book.

Any and all product names referenced within this book are the trademarks of their respective owners. None of these owners have sponsored, authorized, endorsed, or approved this book.

Always read all information provided by the manufacturers' product labels before using their products. The author and publisher are not responsible for claims made by manufacturers.

© **2013**

Manufactured in the United States of America

ENJOY YOUR FREE DOWNLOADS?

PLEASE CLICK HERE TO GIVE ME SOME REVIEWS ON
THE BOOK ...APPRECIATE IT!!

MORE 70 BEST EVER RECIPES EBOOKS REVEALED AT
MY AUTHOR PAGE:-

CLICK HERE TO ACCESS THEM NOW

Introduction

For those looking to serve their families with delicious meals but want to ensure they are providing the healthiest foods are now turning to vegetarian meals. The only difference is that with vegetarian meals, the meals are created using no dairy, no meat, or other animal products including grease or oils. These wonderful meals are not only healthy but delectable as well. Hope you enjoy our vegetarian dinner ideas that you can prepare for your family and guests and be pleased with the compliments you receive.

Chapter 1 - Main Dishes

Pineapple Stir-Fried Rice

Ingredients
3 cups long-grain brown rice
3 tablespoons olive oil
2 sliced onions
4 cups broccoli florets
4 sliced carrots, sliced
2 diced orange bell pepper
6 – 8 sliced scallions
4 diced tomatoes
2 16-ounce cans drained unsweetened pineapple chunks
2 cup light coconut milk
4 tablespoons soy sauce
2 tsp curry powder
4 tsp minced ginger
Cashews for topping

Preparation

Place the rice in a saucepan with 3 cups of water. Bring the rice to a rapid simmer, cover, and cook until the water is completely absorbed around 30 minutes. Just before the rice is done, heat the oil in a skillet and sauté the onion until brown. When the onion is brown add the bell pepper, carrots, and broccoli and turn up heat to medium high. Cook for 3 minutes or until vegetables are tender crisp, then add the pineapple, tomatoes, and scallions and keep stirring frying for 2 minutes longer. Add the rice and stir. Add the curry powder, coconut milk, ginger, and soy sauce. Stir until all ingredients are mixed well. Add cashews on top of each serving. Makes 12 servings.

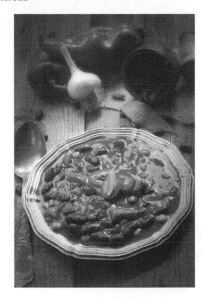

Bean Stew

Ingredients

4 tablespoons olive oil
2 chopped onions
6 minced garlic cloves
4 cups water
4 sliced carrots, peeled and sliced
8 diced celery stalks
1 cup dry red wine
8 cups cooked great northern beans
32 ounces diced tomatoes
1 tsp dried thyme
1 tsp minced fresh rosemary
Salt and pepper to taste
1 cup chopped fresh parsley for garnish

Preparation

Heat the oil in a large pot. Add the onion and sauté until onion is soft. Add the garlic and sauté until both are brown. Add the water, wine, celery, and carrots. Bring to a simmer, cover and cook for 10 minutes. Add the beans, thyme, tomatoes, and rosemary. Stir.

Bring to a simmer, cover, and cook over medium heat for 20 minutes. Add more water if needed. Add ½ cup of parsley, salt, and pepper. Stir to blend, then garnish with more parsley. Makes 12 servings.

Rice and Red Beans

Ingredients

2 ½ cups uncooked brown rice
4 tablespoons olive oil
2 sliced onions
8 minced garlic cloves
2 diced green bell pepper
2 16-ounce cans drained red beans
3 cups diced tomatoes
1 1/3 cup sliced pimiento-stuffed green olives
6 sliced scallions
2 tsp dried oregano
1/2 tsp dried thyme
Cayenne pepper to taste
Salt and pepper to taste
1/2 cup chopped cilantro

Preparation

Place the rice in three cups of water and bring to a rapid simmer, lower the heat, cover, and simmer for 30 minutes. About ½ way through cooking the rice, heat the oil and sauté the onion until soft. Add the bell pepper and garlic and sauté until brown. When the rice is done, add to the sauté pan along with the other ingredients except for the cilantro, salt, and pepper. Cook for 5 minutes and then add the seasoning and cilantro. Makes 12 servings.

Quinoa with Edamame and Oranges

Ingredients

2 cups raw rinsed quinoa
2 tablespoon olive oil
2 cup frozen edamame (thawed)

Samantha Michaels

2 medium cut in strips red bell pepper
12 sliced stalks boy choy
6 sliced scallions
2 tsp dark sesame oil
3 tablespoons teriyaki
2 tsp grated fresh ginger
pepper to taste
4 mandarin oranges in sections
1 cup toasted cashew

Preparation

Add the quinoa to 3 cups of water in a saucepan, bring to a boil, and then lower heat. Cover and simmer around 20 minutes until water is completely absorbed. Heat oil in a pan, add edamame and bell pepper, and stir fry for 3 minutes. Add the scallions and boy choy, cook for 2 minutes. Add the cooked quinoa and sesame oil. Stir. Season to taste with pepper, ginger, and teriyaki sauce. Add the orange sections and cashews. Makes 8 to 12 servings.

Curried Chickpeas

Ingredients

2 tablespoon olive oil
2 chopped onions
4 minced garlic cloves
4 16-ounce cans chickpeas
(drained)
12 ounces frozen green beans
3 tsp garam masala
1 tsp turmeric
1 tsp ground cumin
4 teaspoons grated ginger
4 diced tomatoes
2 tablespoon lemon juice
1/2 cup minced cilantro
Salt to taste

Preparations

Heat oil in a skillet. Add the onion and sauté until soft. Add the garlic and sauté until the onion is brown. Add the green beans, chickpeas, tomatoes, seasonings, lemon juice, and ¼ cup water. Bring to a simmer and cook for 10 minutes stirring often. The mixture should be moist but not think like soup. Add more water if needed. Stir in the cilantro and salt, stir gently. Makes 8 to 12 servings.

Skillet Black Beans

Ingredients

8 potatoes
3 tablespoons olive oil
2 chopped onions
4 minced garlic cloves
2 diced green bell peppers
2 16 oz can diced tomatoes
4 16 oz cans black beans
4 tsp ground cumin
juice of 2 limes
12 corn tortillas cut into strips
Salt to taste

Preparation

Cook potatoes until firm in microwave or oven. Peel, cube, and set aside. Heat oil and sauté onion until soft. Add the bell pepper and garlic, sauté until the onion is brown. Add the cumin, black beans, and tomatoes. Bring to a simmer, cover, and cook 10 minutes. Stir in the potatoes, tortillas, and lime juice, cook until heated thoroughly. Add salt to taste. Makes 8 to 12 servings.

Chickpea Almond Curry

Ingredients

Sauce:

2 minced garlic cloves
1 tsp sea salt

Samantha Michaels

5 tablespoons lime juice
28 oz coconut milk
½ cup almond butter
1 tablespoon tamari
3 tablespoons chopped ginger
3 tsp red curry paste
¼ tsp crushed red pepper flakes

Chickpea Mixture:

8 cups cooked chickpeas
4 cups quartered zucchini
1 ½ cup green onion
4 tablespoons chopped basil

Preparation

Preheat oven to 400 degrees Fahrenheit. While oven is heating, prepare the sauce. In a blender add the garlic, salt, coconut milk, lime juice, tamari, almond butter, curry paste, and tamari. Puree. Put the sauce in a baking dish and stir in the pepper flakes. Add the zucchini, chickpeas, and green onions. Stir until well blended. Cover the baking pan with foil and bake 35 minutes. Remove the foil and continue baking for another 10 minutes. Makes 8 servings.

Paella

2 packages Vegan Chicken strips
16 oz saffron rice
4 cups water
2 tablespoons extra virgin olive oil
3 tsp minced garlic
1 ½ tsp paprika
2 large cans diced tomatoes
15 oz jar marinated artichoke hearts
2 cups sliced roasted red peppers
2 cups sliced snap peas
1 cup white wine
1 tsp salt
½ tsp cracked pepper

Preparation

Bring 2 cups of water to a rapid boil over high heat and then add the rice. Stir for 1 minute, reduce heat, and cook for 20 minutes. Remove from heat and fluff. Set aside with cover on to keep warm. In a skillet, place the olive oil and Vegan chicken strips. Cook around 2 minutes or until the strips are light brown, turn, and brown the other side. Remove from heat and chop into pieces. Set aside and keep warm. To the skillet add the paprika and onion, sauté for 30 seconds. Add the rest of the ingredients and cook on medium heat for around 5 minutes. On a serving platter, place the rice, then the strips, and last the tomato mixture. Makes around 15 servings.

Vegan Shepherd's Pie

Ingredients

Top Layer
10 medium cubed potatoes
1 cup Vegan mayonnaise
1 cup non dairy milk
½ cup olive oil
6 tablespoons vegan cream cheese
4 tsp salt
Bottom layer
2 tablespoon vegetable oil
2 chopped yellow onions
4 chopped carrots
6 chopped stalks celery
1 frozen peas
2 chopped tomatoes
2 minced garlic cloves
28 oz of Vegan ground beef
1 cup shredded vegan Cheddar cheese

Preparation

Cook the potatoes in a pot of water until tender around 30 minutes and then drain. Place the potatoes in a large bowl and add the olive oil, milk, cream cheese, and salt. Mash until smooth and set aside.

Preheat oven to 400 degrees Fahrenheit and grease a large backing dish. In a large skillet over medium heat, heat the oil, and add the carrots, onion, frozen peas, celery, and tomatoes. Cook around 10 minutes until the veggies are soft. Add the garlic. Reduce the heat and crumble the vegan ground beef into the skillet. Cook and stir until meat substitute is hot, usually around 5 minutes. Place the meat mixture in the bottom of the baking dish, spreading to cover the bottom of the pan. Smooth the potato mixture on the top of the meat mixture. Sprinkle with the cheese. Bake around 20 minutes until cheese is melted. Makes 12 servings.

Eggplant Lasagna

Ingredients

1 sliced eggplant
28 oz vegetable pasta sauce
12 oz sliced goat cheese

Preparation

Preheat oven to 350 degrees Fahrenheit. Grease or use cooking spray on a baking dish. Place 1/4 of the sliced eggplant in the bottom of the baking dish in a single layer. Pour ¼ of the sauce over the eggplant. Add around ¼ of the cheese over the sauce. Repeat the layers until all ingredients have been used and end with the cheese. Bake for around 45 minutes to 1 hour until the cheese has melted. Makes 6 servings.

Potato Stir-Fry

Ingredients

1/2 cup cooking oil
8 dried Chile peppers
2 tablespoon cumin seeds
4 tsp split black lentils
1 tsp mustard seeds
2 sprigs curry leaves
2 pounds cubed potatoes
1 tsp red pepper

1 tsp ground cumin
Salt to taste

Preparation

In a large skillet heat the oil. Add the lentils, cumin seeds, Chile peppers, and cook until the seeds start to splutter. Add the curry leaves and cook for 30 seconds. Add the potatoes and stir. Season with salt. Cook for around 20 minutes until the potatoes are tender. Sprinkle the top with cumin powder and pepper and cook for 3 more minutes. Makes 8 servings.

Cornmeal-Crusted Black Bean Burger

Ingredients

30 oz drained black beans
2 vegan egg substitutes
1 cup chopped red bell pepper
2 tablespoon chopped cilantro
2 tsp chili powder
1 tsp ground cumin
1 tsp garlic powder
2/3 cup cornmeal
4 tablespoon extra virgin olive oil
A tad of hot sauce to taste

Preparation

In a large bowl, add the black beans, cilantro, egg, bell pepper, cumin, chili powder, hot sauce, and garlic powder. Mix with your hands until thoroughly blended. Cover the bowl and place in refrigerator overnight. When ready to use, shape into 3 inch burgers. Place the cornmeal in a shallow dish and press the burgers into the cornmeal, turn, and repeat. Heat the oil in a large skill. Cook the burgers for 8 minutes on each side. Makes 10 burgers.

Samantha Michaels

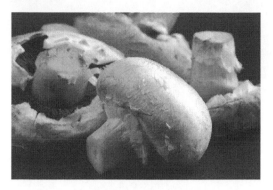

Grilled Stuffed Portobello Mushroom Caps

Ingredients

8 large Portobello mushrooms
4 tsp olive oil
1 cup herb and cooking crème
1 cup quartered grape tomatoes
4 tablespoons Vegan shredded cheese
2 sliced green onions

Preparation

Heat the grill to medium heat. Prepare the mushroom caps by removing the stems and the gills. Brush the caps with oil and grill for 2 minutes on each side. On a foil covered baking sheet, place the mushrooms caps with the rounded sides down. Fill the caps with the rest of the ingredients. Grill for around 7 minutes or until filling is completely warm. Makes 8 servings.

Portobello Mushroom Burger

Ingredients

16 diced plum tomatoes
2/3 cup chopped basil
1/2 cup shredded vegan Parmesan cheese
2 tablespoon balsamic vinegar
4 minced garlic cloves
2 tsp olive oil

4 Portobello mushroom caps
4 tablespoons shredded vegan Cheddar cheese (optional)
2 Kaiser rolls, split
Salt & pepper to taste

Preparation

In a bowl, mix together the basil, tomatoes, parmesan cheese, garlic, olive oil, vinegar, salt, and pepper. Place in refrigerator and allow to sit for 2 hours. This lets the flavors blend. Preheat grill or skillet and lightly oil. Grill the mushroom caps until hot on both sides for 15 minutes. Place the tomato mixture inside the caps. Grill another 15 minutes until thoroughly heated. Add the cheddar cheese and grill until cheese is melted. Makes 4 burgers.

Chapter 2 - Chili's and Stews

Black Bean Chili

Ingredients

3 sweet potatoes
2 tablespoons virgin olive oil
1 cup chopped onion
2 minced garlic cloves
1 diced bell pepper
48 oz cooked black beans
28 oz diced tomatoes
16 oz crushed tomatoes
1 chopped mild green Chile
2 tsp ground cumin
1 tsp oregano
¼ cup minced cilantro
3 sliced scallions
Salt and pepper to taste

Preparation

Bake the sweet potatoes until just firm. Cool, peel, dice, and set aside. Heat the oil in a large pan, sauté the onion and garlic until the onion is brown. Add the rest of the ingredients except for the sweet potatoes, cilantro, scallions, salt and pepper. Bring to a simmer and cook for 15 minutes. Cover and cook another 15 minutes. Add the sweet potatoes and cook for another 15 minutes until veggies are tender. Add the cilantro, scallions, salt, and pepper. Stir gently. Makes around 10 servings.

Hominy Chili

Ingredients

1 1/2 tablespoons olive oil
1 chopped onion
2 minced garlic cloves
1 cut into strips red bell pepper

2 diced sweet potatoes
16-ounce can Great Northern beans
16-ounce can kidney beans
28-ounce can white hominy
16-ounce can diced tomatoes
1 cup frozen corn kernels
1 chopped chili pepper
2 tsp ground cumin
1 tsp dried oregano
1/4 cup chopped cilantro
Salt and dried red pepper flakes to taste
Sliced avocado for garnish

Preparation

In a large pot, sauté the onion until soft. Add the garlic and sauté until the onion is brown. Add 2 cups of water, sweet potatoes, and bell pepper. Bring to a simmer, reduce heat, cover and cook for around 15 minutes until sweet potato is tender. Add the chilies, tomatoes, hominy, oregano, and cumin. Simmer for 20 minutes. Add the cilantro and salt to taste. Add red pepper flakes to taste. Makes around 12 servings.

Moroccan Vegetable Stew

Ingredients

3 tablespoons olive oil
4 chopped onions
4 cubed potatoes
4 cups cubed butternut squash
4 chopped carrots
28 oz diced tomatoes
4 tsp ground cumin
1 tsp ground turmeric
30 oz chickpeas
1 cup couscous
Red pepper flakes, salt, and pepper to taste
Parsley to garnish

Preparation

Heat the oil in a large pot, sauté the onions until brown. Add the potatoes, squash, tomatoes, carrots, and a bit of water to cover. Bring to a simmer, and then add the seasonings. Stir gently, cover, and cook for 45 minutes. Add the chickpeas, along with the red pepper flakes, salt, and pepper to taste. Simmer for another 15 minutes on low heat. Place the couscous in a dish and add 2 cups of water. Let stand for 10 minutes covered, fluff. When ready to serve, place a ladle full of the couscous in the bowl and then add the soup. Makes 12 servings.

Borscht

Ingredients

2 tablespoon olive oil
6 minced garlic cloves
2 chopped onions
6 tablespoons olive oil
4 finely chopped carrots
2 chopped green bell pepper
6 diced beets (include greens)
2 cans whole peeled tomatoes
1 cup diced tomatoes
4 quartered potatoes
2 cups shredded Swiss chard
4 cups vegetable broth
8 cups water
4 tablespoons dried dill weed
32 oz silken tofu
Salt and pepper to taste

Preparation

Heat 1 tablespoon of olive oil in a skillet, sauté the onion until soft around 5 minutes, and set aside. Heat 3 tablespoons of oil in a large pot; add the beets, bell pepper, carrots, celery, potatoes, Swiss chard, tomatoes, and onion mixture. Cook until the chard begins to wilt around 6 minutes. Add the water, broth, dill weed, salt, and pepper, stir, bring to a boil. Reduce heat and simmer 1 hour. Strain ½ the beets and place in a blender. Fill the pitcher about halfway. Pulse until you have a puree. Add the tofu and puree until smooth. Stir the tofu mixture into the pot and simmer for 1 hour. Makes around 15 servings.

Vegan Chili

Ingredients

24 oz crumbled vegan ground beef
30 oz tomato sauce
2 cups water
2 chopped onions
6 minced garlic cloves
2 tablespoon vegan Worcestershire sauce
2 tsp liquid smoke
4 tsp chili powder
¼ tsp black pepper
2 tsp dry mustard
2 tsp salt
¼ red pepper flakes

Preparation

In a large soup pot add all ingredients and stir. Cook on low heat for 30 minutes or until hot. Makes 8 to 12 servings.

Mexican Stew

Ingredients

10 peeled & cubed potatoes
4 chopped carrots
2 chopped celery stalks
9 cups water
8 cubes vegetable bouillon
2 tablespoons olive oil
2 diced onions
8 minced garlic cloves
2 tablespoons chili powder
2 tablespoons cumin
3 tablespoons seasoned salt
2 cans drained hominy

Samantha Michaels

2 cans diced tomatoes
Salt and pepper to taste

Preparation

Place the celery, carrots, and potatoes in a large pot and enough water to cover and salt. Bring to a boil and cook for 10 minutes until a tad tender. Drain and set aside. In a pot add 4 ½ cups water and the bouillon cubes and bring to a boil. Cook until cubes are completely dissolved. Remove from heat and set aside. Heat the oil in skillet, sauté garlic and onion until soft. Season with seasoned salt, cumin, and chili powder. Add the potato mixture and cook for 2 minutes. Add the rest of the water and the bouillon mixture, tomatoes, chilies, and hominy. Bring to a boil, reduce heat, cook for 45 minutes. Season to taste. Makes 15 servings.

Chapter 3 - Casseroles

Vegetable Pot Pie

Ingredients

8 potatoes
2 tablespoons virgin olive oil
1 chopped onion
3 cups diced vegetables such as peas, cauliflower, broccoli, mushrooms, or your favorites. You should have one cup of each veggie
2 tablespoons flour
1 cup vegetable stock
½ cup nutritional yeast
1 ½ tablespoons seasoning blend
1 tsp dried thyme
¼ cup minced parsley
2 9-inch pie crusts
1 cup bread crumbs
Salt and pepper to taste

Preparation

Bake or microwave the potatoes until soft. When cook, peel, dice, and mash. Only mash about ½ of the potatoes. Set aside. Preheat oven to 350 degrees Fahrenheit. Heat oil in large skillet, sauté the onion until brown. Add the vegetables, a small bit of water, and cook until veggies are tender around 5 minutes. Add a tad of flour to the skillet and pour in the stock. Add the yeast. Cook for 2 minutes constantly stirring until the liquid becomes thick. Add the mashed and diced potatoes. Stir gently. Add the parsley, thyme, and seasoning blend. Pour into the pie crusts. Sprinkle the bread crumbs over both pies. Bake for 40 minutes or until crust is golden. Makes 2 pies.

Vegan Casserole

Ingredients

10 peeled potatoes
2 crushed garlic cloves
2 minced garlic cloves
2 chopped celery stalks
2 bunches chopped parsley
16 whole black peppercorns
2 chopped onions
1 bay leaf
2 tablespoons light miso paste
8 tablespoons olive oil
1 ½ cups chopped red onion
1 pound sliced mushrooms
2 pound2 crumbled firm tofu
8 tablespoons barbecue sauce
4 tablespoon vegan gravy mix
2 tsp paprika
2 tablespoon tamari
2 cups fresh corn kernels
2 cups chopped spinach
1/4 cup whole wheat flour
2 cubes vegetable bouillon

Preparation

Preheat oven to 400 degrees Fahrenheit. Peel and quarter the potatoes. Place in a large pot with enough water to cover. Add the bay leaf, onion, parsley, celery, and garlic. Bring to a boil, cover and simmer for 20 minutes. To make the filling, Sauté the onion and garlic in 1 tablespoon of oil for 1 minute. Add the mushrooms and sauté for 2 minutes. Crumble the tofu into the skillet and sauté while blending well. Add the gravy mix, barbeque sauce, thyme, tamari, and mix well. Sauté for 20 minutes. Place the potatoes in a large bowl while setting aside 7 cups of the stock. Add the oil, miso, and 2 cups of the potato stock a few at a time. Mash the potatoes as you add the stock. Do not get to moist as this is the crust. Add the spinach and corn to the filling mixture, then place in a greased baking dish. Spread the potato crust. Bake for 40 minutes or until crust is golden brown. While baking, in a skillet make the gravy using the potato sock and the gravy mix. Spoon gravy over casserole. Makes 8 to 12 servings.

Butternut Squash Casserole

Ingredients

6 cups cooked & mashed butternut squash
1 cup white sugar
1 cup packed brown sugar
½ cup melted vegan margarine
16 oz can crushed pineapple with juice
2 tsp ground cinnamon
2 tsp vanilla extract
¼ tsp ground nutmeg
2/3 cup chopped walnuts

Preparation

Preheat oven to 325 degrees Fahrenheit. Grease a baking dish and set aside. Combine all the ingredients except for the walnuts in a bowl and mix well. Pour into the baking dish. Sprinkle with the walnuts and bake for 40 minutes. Makes 12 servings.

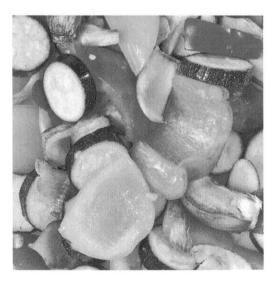

Layered Vegetable Casserole

Ingredients

2 eggplants

2 thinly sliced zucchini,
56 oz of pasta sauce
Bean filling

Preparation

Peel and cut the eggplant into ¼ inch pieces. Bake in the oven until the eggplant pieces are slightly shriveled. Remove and place on plate, set aside. Preheat oven to 425 degrees Fahrenheit. Grease a baking dish. Add a layer of the pasta sauce to the baking dish, place eggplant slices over the sauce, then a layer of bean filling, and then zucchini. Drizzle a little more sauce then repeat the process. Spread the last bit of sauce over the top of the last bit of zucchini. Bake for 30 minutes. Makes 12 servings.

Sweet Potato Casserole

Ingredients

4 tsp vegetable oil
1 ½ cup chopped onion
4 tsp grated gingerroot
4 minced garlic cloves
16 oz can tomato sauce
1 cup water
1 cup creamy peanut butter
2 tsp ground cumin
2 tsp ground coriander
4 large cans sweet potatoes
2 tablespoon chopped cilantro

Preparation

Preheat the oven to 375 degrees Fahrenheit. Grease a baking dish. Heat the oil in a skillet, sauté the onion for 5 minutes. Add the garlic and gingerroot and sauté for 1 minute. Add the cumin, peanut butter, water, tomato sauce, and coriander, stir until well blended and smooth. Cook for 2 minutes, constantly stirring. Add the sweet potatoes and mash the potatoes until blended. Spoon into the baking dish. Bake for 39 minutes. Makes 12 servings.

Pasta and Bean Casserole

Ingredients

2 16-oz packages pasta
4 tablespoons olive oil
2 diced onions
6 minced garlic cloves
1 chopped green bell pepper
1 chopped red bell pepper
2 14.5-oz cans diced tomatoes
2 15-oz cans garbanzo beans
2 tsp basil
2 tsp dried oregano
2 tsp ground paprika
2 tsp ground cumin
2 tsp ground coriander
salt and pepper to taste
1 cup shredded vegan mozzarella cheese

Preparation

Preheat oven to 350 degrees Fahrenheit. Grease a baking dish. Cook pasta as directed on the package, drain, and set aside. Heat oil in a skillet, sauté onion until soft. Add the garlic and peppers and cook for 2 minutes. Add the beans and tomatoes. Add the cumin, coriander, oregano, basil, salt and pepper. Simmer for 5 minutes. Remove from heat and add the pasta. Stir gently. Pour into the baking dish, spread the cheese, and bake for 30 minutes or until cheese is melted. Makes 12 servings.

Millet

Ingredients

2 cups uncooked millet
1 cup non dairy milk powder
11 cups hot water
1 1/3 cups chopped dates
1 cup flaked coconut
2 tsp vanilla extract

Preparation

Preheat oven to 350 degrees Fahrenheit. Combine the dates, hot water, milk powder, millet, coconut, and vanilla in a baking dish. Bake for 30 minutes, remove, and stir. Return to the oven and bake for another 30 minutes. Makes 16 servings.

Mashed Potato & Vegetable Enchiladas

Ingredients

½ head broccoli florets
4 oz whole button mushrooms
1/2 chopped zucchini
1 cup chopped carrots
1/8 cup olive oil
1 ½ cups water
½ cup non dairy milk
½ package instant potato flakes
6 oz package corn tortillas
1 ½ cups enchilada sauce
4 oz vegan shredded Cheddar cheese
Salt and pepper to taste

Preparation

Preheat oven to 425 degrees Fahrenheit. In a bowl, mix the carrots, zucchini, broccoli, and mushrooms. Drizzle olive oil over the veggies and season. Place the veggies in a baking dish. Bake for 15 minutes, stir, and bake for another 15 minutes. Remove and lower the temperature to 350 degrees Fahrenheit. In a large pot, bring the milk and water to a boil. Remove from heat and add the potato flakes. Let stand for 2 minutes. Stir in the vegetables. In a skillet, heat each tortilla, then dip in the enchilada sauce. Add a spoonful of the potato mixture to each tortilla along with 2 tablespoons of cheese. Roll the tortilla and place seam down in the baking dish. Pour the rest of the sauce over the top and sprinkle with cheese. Bake for 20 minutes. Makes 6 servings.

Chapter 4 - Tortilla Dishes

Tortilla Casserole

Ingredients

2 16-oz cans pinto beans
2 16-oz cans black beans
2 16-oz cans crushed tomatoes
2 4-oz cans chopped mild green chilies
1 hot minced chili
4 cups thawed frozen corn kernels
4 minced scallions
2 tsp ground cumin
2 tsp dried oregano
20 corn tortillas
3 cups grated nondairy cheddar cheese
Salsa and vegan sour cream for topping

Preparation

Preheat oven to 400 degrees Fahrenheit. In a large bowl, combine the beans, cumin, oregano, chilies, corn, scallions, and tomatoes, blend well. Grease a baking dish. Then layer the ingredients like: tortillas, bean mixture, cheese, repeat until you run out of ingredients. Bake for 15 minutes or until cheese is bubbly. Top with salsa and sour cream. Makes 12 servings.

Vegetable Burritos

Ingredients

16 flour tortillas
3 tablespoons olive oil
3 sliced onions
4 cups broccoli florets
2 red bell pepper, cut into strips
2 diced zucchini
2 diced tomatoes
2 minced hot chilies

2 4-oz can chopped green chilies
2 15- to 16-oz cans refried beans
2 tsp chili powder
2 tsp ground cumin
2 cups grated non-dairy cheese
Salsa or picante sauce

Preparation

Allow the tortillas to warm to room temperature. Heat oil and sauté onion until soft. Add the broccoli and pepper strips. Do not stir. Cook for 5 minutes. Add the tomato, zucchini, chilies, and stir well. Cover and cook for 7 minutes or until veggies are tender. Drain off any liquid. Place the refried beans in a sauce pan and add a small amount of water. Stir in the cumin and chili powder. Cook until heated. On the tortilla shell add the refried beans, then the veggies, and last cheese. Roll up and place on plate with seam side down. Serve with salsa or picante sauce. Makes 8 servings.

Black Bean Tostadas

Ingredients

16 corn tortillas
Bean topping
2 tablespoon olive oil
2 chopped onions
4 minced garlic cloves
4 15-to 16-oz cans black beans
4 sliced scallions
2 sliced green chili peppers
Salt and pepper to taste
4 tsp ground cumin
Garnishes
Shredded lettuce
Salsa
Vegan sour cream

Preparation

Preheat oven to 375 degrees Fahrenheit. Place the tortilla shells on a baking sheet and bake for 10 minutes or until crisp. Remove and place on a platter. Heat oil in skillet and sauté the onion and garlic until onion is brown around 5 minutes. Add the rest of the ingredients except for the beans, along with a ½ cup of water. Simmer. While simmering, mash a few of the beans so the liquid becomes thick. Place in serving dish. Let the guests layer their tostados. Makes 16 tostados.

Cauliflower Tacos

Ingredients

Roasted Cauliflower:

2 heads of cauliflower divided into florets
4 tablespoons olive oil
1 tsp salt

Chick Peas:

2 15-oz can chick peas
2 tablespoon olive oil
2 tsp salt
1/2 tsp chili powder
1/2 tsp ground cumin
1/2 tsp ground oregano

Cilantro-Pepita Pesto:

4 cups cilantro leaves
2/3 cup toasted pumpkin seeds
2 garlic cloves, cut in half
4 tablespoons chopped jalapeño chiles
4 tablespoons lime juice
1 tsp salt
1/2 cup olive oil
16 corn tortillas

Preparation

Preheat oven to 425 degrees to Fahrenheit. In a large bowl, place the cauliflower and drizzle with 4 tablespoons oil. Sprinkle with salt. Stir and place on a baking sheet. Bake for 15 minutes or until cauliflower is tender. Mix all the chick pea ingredients. Spread in a baking dish. Bake for 15 minutes or until chickpeas are brown and crispy. In a blender add all the pesto ingredients except for the oil. As the blender is running on low, slowly ad the oil. Half way through stir and then start again. Place pesto in bowl. Add 1 tablespoon of the pesto on each tortilla, add ½ cup cauliflower and 1 tablespoon of the chick peas. Makes 16 tacos.

Vegan Quesadillas

Ingredients

Vegan wraps
1 chopped tomato
1 chopped green pepper
1 chopped onion
1 can black beans
Lettuce

Preparation

Chop all the veggies and place in separate bowls. Open and drain the can of beans and place in a bowl. Let everyone make their own quesadillas.

Farmer's Market Vegetarian Quesadillas

Ingredients

1 cup chopped red bell pepper
1cup chopped zucchini
1 cup chopped yellow squash
1 cup chopped red onion
1 cup chopped mushrooms
2 tablespoon olive oil
cooking spray
12 (9 inch) whole wheat tortillas
1 1/2 cups vegan shredded Cheddar cheese

Preparation

In a skillet add the squash, onion, mushrooms, zucchini, red pepper, and olive oil. Cook over medium high heat for 7 minutes or until veggies are tender. Remove veggies from pan. In the same pan, place one tortilla and sprinkle with cheese, add some of the veggie mixture, and sprinkle again with cheese, then top with another tortilla. Cook and turn until both sides are golden brown around 2 minutes per side. Cut each quesadilla into 8 triangles. Makes 6 quesadillas.

Vegan Enchiladas

Ingredients

Sauce:

4 pounds fresh tomatillos
2 chopped white onions
4 chopped garlic cloves
2 chopped jalapeño
4 cups vegetable stock
1 cup chopped cilantro
Salt and pepper to taste

Enchiladas:

4 cups diced butternut squash
4 tablespoons olive oil
Salt and pepper to taste
2 chopped onions
4 minced shallots
4 cups thinly sliced shiitake caps
4 cups frozen corn kernels
4 cups finely chopped Tuscan kale
2 cup canola oil
24 corn tortillas

Crema:

2 cups raw cashews

4 tablespoons lime juice
2 tsp white vinegar
2 tsp smoked paprika
1 tsp salt

Preparation

In a bowl, cover the cashews with hot water and let stand for around 2 hours. Drain and place in a food processor. To the cashews add paprika, vinegar, lime juice, salt, and ½ cup of water. Puree until smooth. To make the sauce, in a pan add the onion, jalapeno, tomatillos, garlic, and stock, bring to a simmer. Cook over medium heat around 15 minutes or until veggies are tender. Place this in a food processor and add the cilantro and puree until smooth. Add salt and pepper. Preheat oven to 400 degrees Fahrenheit. In a baking dish place the squash and 1 tablespoon of olive oil. Roast for 15 minutes. Remove squash, lower temperature to 375 degrees. In a skillet, sauté the onion, shallots with 2 tablespoons of olive oil until brown around 5 minutes. Add the shitake and cook 6 minutes. Add the kale and corn and cook another 5 minutes. Add the squash. In another skillet, heat the canola oil. Dip the tortilla in the pan and turn once. Add the filling equally into the tortilla and place them in a baking dish. Add remaining sauce on top. Make 25 minutes. Makes 12 servings.

Tortilla Stew

Ingredients

2 19-oz cans enchilada sauce
3 cups water
2 cube vegetable bouillon
1 tsp garlic powder
1/2 tsp chili powder
1/2 tsp ground cumin
2 15-oz cans pinto beans
1 16-oz can diced tomatoes
2 cups frozen corn
1 cup diced vegetarian chicken substitute
8 torn into strips corn tortillas
2 tablespoon chopped cilantro

Salt and pepper to taste

Preparation

In a pan, mix the water and enchilada sauce. Dissolve the bouillon cube in the mixture and add garlic powder, cumin, and chile powder. Bring to a boil, reduce heat, and simmer. Stir in the corn, beans, and tomatoes. Simmer until well heated. Stir in the tortillas and vegan chicken. Cook until heated thoroughly. Stir in the cilantro, salt and pepper. Makes 8 servings.

Seitan and Black Bean Burritos

Ingredients

6 tablespoons olive oil
2 chopped onions
10 chopped green onions
4 minced garlic cloves
4 minced chili peppers
2 chopped red bell peppers
16 oz package seitan
2 15-oz can black beans
2 16-oz can diced tomatoes
6 cups cooked white rice
6 tablespoons chopped cilantro
2 18-oz bottles barbecue sauce
20 flour tortillas

Preparation

In a pan heat oil and sauté onions, chili peppers, and bell peppers until onions are translucent around 5 minutes. Add the seitan and sauté for 5 more minutes. Add the tomatoes and beans and heat thoroughly. In a bowl, add this mixture to the cooked rice, 1 cup of barbecue sauce, and cilantro. Mix well. Place tortillas on flat surface and place around ¾ cup of mixture in the center of each one. Wrap the tortillas. Place the burritos in a baking dish, pour the rest of the barbeque sauce on top, and bake for 35 minutes. Makes 20 burritos

Chapter 5 - Pizzas

Asparagus & Spinach Pizza

Ingredients

12 asparagus spears
4 oz baby spinach
1 12.3-ounce firm silken tofu
1 tsp salt
One 12-oz pizza crust
1/3 cup cut into strips sun-dried tomatoes
1 cup nondairy mozzarella cheese

Preparation

Preheat oven to 425 degrees Fahrenheit. Cut the asparagus into 1 inch pieces and place in a cover pan with a little bit of water. Steam until the asparagus is bright green. Add the spinach and steam until wilted around 1 minute. Drain and set aside. Puree the tofu in a food processor with salt. Spread the tofu on the pizza crust. Scatter the spinach and asparagus evenly over the top and then add the tomatoes. Bake for 12 minutes or until crust is golden brown. Makes one pizza.

Veggie Pizza

Ingredients

1 link sliced vegan sausage
1 cut into strips red bell pepper
1 cup broccoli florets
1 sliced zucchini
1 1/2 tablespoons olive oil
2/3 cup pizza sauce
1 12-oz pizza crust
1 cup grated nondairy cheese
Dried basil

Preparation

Preheat the oven to 425 degrees Fahrenheit. In a bowl, stir together the zucchini, broccoli, sausage, and bell pepper. Place in a baking dish that has been lightly oiled. Place in a hot oven. Evenly spread the pizza sauce on the crust. Sprinkle with cheese. Cut the pizza into 6 to 8 slices. Remove the veggies and place the crust in the oven for 10 minutes. Stir the veggies. Place the veggies back in the oven and bake for 15 minutes. Place the veggies on the pizza crust evenly. Makes 1 pizza.

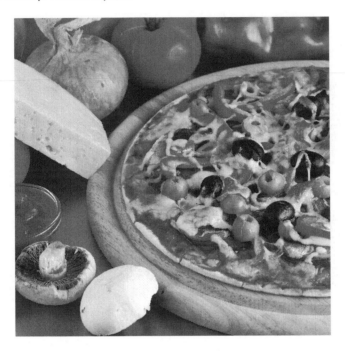

Margherita Pizza

Ingredients

Sauce:

1 tablespoon olive oil
1/2 cup minced onion
3 minced garlic cloves
1/2 tsp dried thyme
1/2 tsp dried basil
1/4 tsp ground fennel
1/4 tsp red pepper flakes

Salt and black pepper
1 cup chopped roasted red bell peppers
1 15-oz can diced tomatoes
1 tablespoon capers
1 tablespoon agave nectar

Dough:

1 cup warm water
1 tsp agave nectar
2 1/4 tsp active yeast
2 cups all-purpose flour
1/2 cup whole-wheat pastry flour
1 tablespoon nutritional yeast
2 tsp salt
2 tablespoons plus 1 tsp olive oil

Toppings:

6 plum tomatoes, cut into 1/4-inch slices
2 cups shredded vegan mozzarella cheese
1 cup finely chopped basil

Preparation

In a bowl combine the agave nectar, ¾ cup warm water, and yeast. Set aside until bubbly. In another bowl, combine flours, herbs, salt, and nutritional yeast. Add the first yeast mixture along with 2 tablespoons olive oil. Stir. Add the other ¼ cup of water. Knead 10 minutes and shape into a ball. Oil a large bowl and place the dough in the bowl. Roll to coat the ball. Cover and set aside for 1 hour. To make the sauce, heat the oil in pan, add the herbs, red pepper flakes, garlic and onion. Add salt and pepper to taste, sauté 5 minutes. Add the rest of the ingredients and bring to a boil, reduce heat and simmer 20 minutes. Preheat oven to 475 degrees Fahrenheit. Make two balls of dough and roll out dough 2 12 inch rounds. Top each pizza with the sauce, tomato slices, cheese and other toppings. Bake 10 minutes.

Fast Vegan Pizza

Ingredients

4 cups chopped eggplant
2 cups tomato sauce
tad of crushed red peppers
tad of sugar
2 pizza dough's
2 cups spinach
1 sliced red bell pepper
1 cup artichoke hearts
1/2 cup sliced red onions
1/2 quartered black olives

Preparation

In a skillet bring 2 tablespoons of water to a simmer. Add the eggplant until all water has evaporated around 3 minutes. Add the red pepper, sugar, and tomato sauce. Cook around 7 minutes until eggplant is soft. Set aside to cool. Preheat oven to 500 degrees Fahrenheit. Press the pizza dough into your pizza pan, cover with the sauce, top with black olives, spinach, artichoke hearts, onions, and bell peppers. Bake for 10 minutes. Makes 2 pizzas.

No Cheese Pizza

Ingredients

Crust:

1 package active dry yeast
1 tsp sugar
1 cup warm water
2 1/2 cups white flour

Pizza Toppings:

1 oz fresh basil
4 tablespoons olive oil
3 crushed garlic cloves

3 tablespoons ketchup
2 tablespoons pine nuts
1 tablespoon lemon juice
3 sliced plum tomatoes
2 cups sliced mushrooms
1 sliced onion

Preparation

Mix water, sugar, yeast, and let stand 10 minutes. When it begins to bubble add the flour and mix well. Place the mixture in a greased bowl, cover with a damp towel, and allow to rise 1 hour. Punch the dough and pat into a pizza pan. Bake in 450 degree Fahrenheit preheated oven for 7 minutes. Turn the oven down to 350 degrees Fahrenheit. In a blender add garlic, basil, pine nuts, ketchup, olive oil, and lemon juice. Blend until smooth. Spread over the pizza crust. Add mushrooms, tomatoes, and onions or other veggies. Bake for 10 minutes. Makes 1 pizza.

Alfredo Pizza

Ingredients

Sauce:

6 tablespoon vegan cream
2 tablespoon vegan butter
1 tablespoon nutritional yeast
1 tablespoon wheat flour
1 tablespoon vegan grated parmesan cheese
1 garlic clove
Salt and pepper to taste

Vegan Pesto:

1 ½ cup basil
¼ cup olive oil
1 cup toasted pine nuts
5 garlic cloves
1 tsp salt
1 tsp black pepper

¼ cup vegan grated parmesan

Preparation

For the sauce, in a skillet sauté garlic in vegan butter. Season with salt and pepper. Add the cream and allow to warm. Add the nutritional yeast and flour until mixture becomes thick. Add the parmesan cheese. For the pesto, blend all ingredients in a food processor. Makes 1 pizza.

Aloha Pizza

Ingredients

1 pizza crust
1 cup vegan barbecue sauce
8 round slices pineapple
1 cup vegan chicken
1/2 cup sun dried tomatoes
1 cup vegan Mozzarella cheese
1/2 cup chopped onions

Preparation

Roast the vegan chicken as directed by the package. Set aside. Grill the pineapple rounds. Preheat oven to 425 degrees Fahrenheit. Start making your pizza by layering with cheese, onions, tomatoes, pineapples, and chicken. Bake for 15 minutes. Makes 1 pizza.

White Pan Pizza

Ingredients

2 pizza crusts
3/4 cup plain soy yogurt
1 tablespoon nutritional yeast
1 tablespoon dried parsley
1 tsp onion powder
1/2 tsp garlic powder
1/4 tsp mustard powder
1/4 tsp salt

Samantha Michaels

1/2 lb button mushrooms
1/4 lb shiitake mushrooms
Parsley

Preparation

Preheat oven to 425 degrees Fahrenheit. In a bowl, mix the spices and yogurt until smooth. Prepare the mushrooms and herbs, then set aside. Spread the white sauce on the pizza crusts, sprinkle with mushrooms and bake for 8 minutes or until the crust is golden. Sprinkle with your herbs.

Chapter 6 – Pasta

Chickpeas & Greens Pasta

Ingredients

20 ounces rotini
4 tablespoons olive oil
4 minced garlic cloves
2 cut into strips red bell pepper
20 ounces spinach
6 diced tomatoes
2 16-oz can chickpeas
1 cup sliced olives
2 tsp dried oregano
Salt and pepper to taste

Preparation

Cook the pasta as directed on package, drain, and place in a large bowl. Heat oil in skillet, sauté the bell pepper and garlic until soft around 3 minutes. Add the spinach, cover, and wilt for 30 seconds. Add the oregano, olives, chickpeas, and tomatoes, stir. Cook for 4 minutes. Combine this mixture in the pasta. Toss. Makes 8 to 10 servings.

Roasted Veggies & Pasta

Ingredients

10 ounces spiral pasta
1 eggplant, cut into 1/4-inch-thick slices
1 red bell pepper, cut into 1-inch squares
4 cups small broccoli florets
2 tablespoons virgin olive oil
1/2 sliced red onion
4 sliced garlic cloves
1/3 cup sliced sun-dried tomatoes
1/2 cup olives
1/4 cup minced fresh parsley

1 tablespoon balsamic vinegar or more to taste, optional
Dried red pepper flakes to taste
Salt and freshly ground pepper to taste

Preparation

Preheat the oven to 425 degrees Fahrenheit. Grease a roasting pan. In a bowl, mix the eggplant and bell pepper. Drizzle half the oil over the eggplant and stir. Place in the roasting pan. In the same bowl, mix the garlic, onion, and broccoli and using the rest of the oil drizzle the veggies. Add to the roasting pan and mix gently. Place in the oven and roast for 20 minutes. Cook pasta as directed on package, drain, and pour into a large bowl. Add the vinegar, tomatoes, parsley, and olives. Stir together with vegetables. Add the pasta to the vegetables and toss. Season with salt, pepper, and red pepper flakes. Makes 6 servings.

Pasta Curry

Ingredients

1 lb penne
2 tablespoons olive oil
2 chopped onions
4 minced garlic cloves
2 red bell peppers cut into strips
8 cups cauliflower florets
2 28-oz can diced tomatoes
2 tablespoon curry powder
2 tsp dried basil
2 15-oz can chickpeas
1 cup raisins
4 handfuls of baby spinach
Salt and red pepper flakes to taste

Preparation

Cook the pasta as directed on the package. While the pasta is cooking, heat oil in skillet and sauté onion and garlic until onion is brown. Add the basil, curry powder, bell peppers, tomatoes, and cauliflower. Cook for 15 to 20 minutes until cauliflower is tender.

Add the raisins and chickpeas, simmer for 5 minutes. Add the spinach, cover, and cook until wilted. In a bowl, combine the cauliflower mixture and pasta. Stir in the cilantro, salt, and red pepper flakes. Makes 12 servings.

Penne with Beans

Ingredients

10 ounces chard
10 ounces penne pasta
2 tablespoons virgin olive oil
1 sliced onion
3 minced garlic cloves
1/4 cup water
1 ½ pounds diced tomatoes
1 15-oz can red beans
10 sliced basil leaves
1/3 cup raisins
Salt and pepper to taste

Preparation

Cut the leaves from the chard stems and set aside. Chop the leaves and slice the stems. Rinse well. Bring water to a boil and cook pasta as directed on the package. Heat the oil and sauté garlic and onion until golden brown around 5 minutes. Add the water and the stems, cover and cook until chard wilts around 3 minutes. Stir in the beans, raisins, and tomatoes. Cook around 5 minutes until heated well. Combine the pasta with the sauce in a bowl. Toss well add salt and pepper to taste. Makes 6 servings.

Baked Spaghetti Squash

Ingredients

2 spaghetti squash, halved lengthwise
2 chopped onions
4 tablespoons minced garlic
4 14-oz cans stewed tomatoes
2 tablespoon dried basil

2 cubes vegetable bouillon
salt and pepper to taste
2 15-oz can chopped black olives
2 cups shredded mozzarella cheese
2 cups shredded Parmesan cheese

Preparation

Preheat oven to 325 degrees Fahrenheit. Grease a baking sheet. Place the squash halves with the cut side down on the sheet. Bake 35 minutes, remove, and cool. Using a non stick saucepan, sauté garlic and onion until brown. Stir in the cube, pepper, basil, and tomatoes. Cook for 15 minutes. Remove the strands of squash with a fork. Layer the inside the squash with a spoonful of the sauce, the squash strands, olives, mozzarella cheese. Repeat the layers until the squash is full. Top with parmesan cheese. Bake for 20 minutes. Makes 12 servings.

Zucchini Alfredo

Ingredients

2 12-oz packages uncooked egg noodles
6 tablespoons vegetable oil
4 minced garlic cloves
8 cups shredded zucchini
1 cup non dairy milk
8 oz of cubed vegan cream cheese
1 cup chopped fresh basil
Salt and pepper to taste

Preparation

Bring a pot of salted water to a boil and add egg noodles. Cook for 10 minutes and drain. Heat oil in a skillet and sauté garlic for 2 minutes. Add the zucchini and cook 10 minutes. Add the milk and cream cheese to the skillet and cook until melted. Mix in basil. Season with salt and pepper. Sprinkle with parmesan cheese and serve over the cooked pasta. Makes 12 servings.

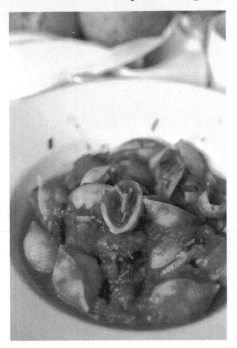

Pesto Polenta Lasagna

Ingredients

2 18 oz packages polenta, cut into 1/4 inch thick slices
1 24 oz jar marinara sauce
1/2 cup pesto
½ cup pine nuts
2 cups shredded vegan mozzarella cheese

Preparation

Preheat oven to 375 degrees Fahrenheit. Grease a baking dish. Add the polenta to the bottom of the baking sheet. Spread a layer of the pest over the top of the polenta. Spoon sauce over the polenta. Repeat until ingredients are gone. Bake for 25 minutes. Top with cheese and pine nuts and broil until cheese is brown. Makes 16 servings.

Samantha Michaels

Sukhothai Pad Thai

Ingredients

1 cup sugar
1 cup distilled white vinegar
1/2 cup soy sauce
4 tablespoons tamarind pulp
2 12-oz package dried rice noodles
1 cup vegetable oil
3 tsp minced garlic
8 egg substitutes
2 12-oz firm tofu cut into ½ strips
3 tablespoons sugar
3 tablespoons salt
3 cups ground peanuts
3 tsp ground dried radish
1 cup chopped fresh chives
2 tablespoon paprika
3 cups fresh bean sprouts
2 lime, cut into wedges

Preparation

In a saucepan, blend soy sauce, vinegar, and tamarind pulp and cook over medium heat. Soak the rice noodles in cold water until soft, then drain. In a skillet warm oil and add the egg substitute and garlic. Stir and scramble. Add the tofu and stir until well blended. Add the noodles and stir until soft. In the sauce, add the sugar and salt. Stir in the radish and peanuts. Remove from heat and add paprika and chives. Serve with the bean sprouts and lime on the side. Makes 16 servings.

Lime Orzo

Ingredients

4 tablespoons olive oil
4 minced garlic cloves
4 cups orzo pasta
2 shredded zucchinis

2 shredded carrots
2 16-oz can stewed tomatoes
2 14-oz can vegetable broth
2 tsp Italian seasoning
2 tsp dried basil leaves
salt and pepper to taste
½ cup chopped green onions
½ cup chopped fresh parsley
4 tsp grated lime zest
4 tablespoons lime juice
1 cup grated Parmesan cheese for topping

Preparation

Heat oil in skillet, add the pasta and garlic. Cook and stir until pasta is a light golden brown, around 5 minutes. Stir in the carrots and zucchini, cook until the vegetables are soft around 2 minutes. Stir in basil, seasoning, broth, and tomatoes. Season with salt and pepper to taste. Reduce heat, cover, simmer around 10 minutes. Stir in the parsley, green onions, lime juice, and lime zest. Remove from heat, serve with parmesan cheese. Makes 8 servings.

Borboletas

Ingredients

2 16-oz package dry bow tie pasta
2 chopped tomatoes
2 chopped cucumbers
8 ounces crumbled feta cheese
½ cup Italian salad dressing
2 tsp dried oregano

Preparation

Bring a pot of salted water to a boil. Place the pasta in the pot and cook for 10 minutes, drain. In a bowl, toss the pasta with the feta cheese, cucumber, tomato, oregano, and Italian dressing. Makes 16 servings.

Samantha Michaels

Spaghetti

Ingredients

2 16-oz package spaghetti
2 cups chopped onion
1 cup chopped celery
2 tsp garlic powder
6 tablespoons vegetable oil
2 26-oz jar spaghetti sauce
2 16-oz can garbanzo beans
2 14.5-oz can diced tomatoes
2 tsp sugar
1 tsp salt
1 tsp dried oregano
1 bay leaf
½ cup grated Parmesan cheese

Preparation

Cook spaghetti according to directions on package. In a skillet, sauté the celery, onion, and garlic powder in oil until onion is tender. Add the spaghetti sauce, tomatoes, beans, bay leaf, salt, oregano, and sugar. Bring to a boil, cover, and simmer for 10 minutes. Remove the bay leaf. Drain the spaghetti and top with sauce and parmesan cheese. Makes 12 servings.

Chapter 7 – Desserts

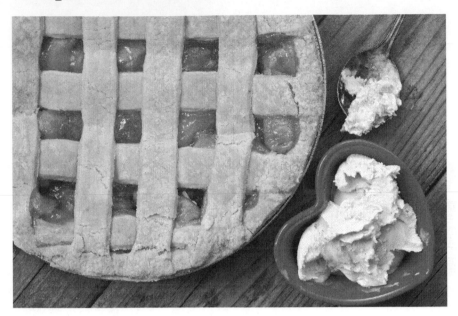

Applesauce Cake

Ingredients

1 ¾ cups whole wheat flour
1/3 cup quick oats
1 tsp baking soda
2 tsp baking powder
2 tsp cinnamon
1/2 tsp cloves
1 tsp nutmeg
1/4 tsp salt
1 tablespoon ground flax seed, beaten with 2 tablespoon water, let sit for 5 minutes
4 cups unsweetened applesauce
1 cup frozen apple juice concentrate
4 tablespoon sunflower seed oil
4 tablespoon lemon juice
2 tsp vanilla

Preparation

Preheat oven to 350 degrees Fahrenheit. Grease a cake with vegetable oil. Combing spices, baking powder, baking soda, oats, and flour in a large bowl. Mix all the wet ingredients together along with the oil and flax seed mixture. Mix the wet and dry ingredients together and stir until well blended. Pour into the cake pan and smooth with a spatula. Bake for 50 minutes. Makes 12 servings.

Blueberry Streusel Cake

Ingredients

3 cups flour
1 1/2 tsp baking powder
1 tsp baking soda
1 tsp salt
3/4 cup white sugar
Zest from one lemon
1 cup orange juice
1 1/4 cup soy milk
1/3 cup oil
1 tablespoon ground flax seed
2 cups blueberries mixed with ½ cup flour
Streusel Topping Ingredients:
3/4 cup flour
1/2 cup sugar
1/3 cup earth balance

Preparation

Preheat oven to 375 degrees Fahrenheit. Grease a cake pan and set aside. Make the topping and set aside by combining all ingredients until crumbly. Using a whisk, combine milk, juice, oil, and ground flax seeds, set aside. Combine the baking powder, flour, baking soda, lemon zest, and salt. Stir the wet ingredients into the dry ingredients until mixed. Fold the blueberries into the batter. Scrape the batter in the baking pan. Sprinkle the topping on top. Bake for 45 minutes until the topping is golden. Makes 12 servings.

Gingerbread

Ingredients

1/4 cup unrefined cane sugar
1/4 cup coconut oil
1 cup light molasses
1/2 cup unsweetened applesauce
1 cup hot water
1 tablespoon ground flaxseeds
1 1/4 cups sorghum flour
1/2 cup arrowroot starch
1/2 cup teff flour
1/4 cup millet flour
2 tsp ground cinnamon
2 tsp ground ginger
2 tsp xanthan gum
1 1/2 tsp baking soda
1/2 tsp ground cloves
1/2 tsp ground nutmeg
1/2 tsp sea salt

Preparation

Preheat oven to 350 degrees Fahrenheit. Grease a baking pan. Place the sugar and oil in a large bowl on medium speed until well combined. Beat in the molasses until well blended. In a small bowl or measuring cup add the flax seeds and water. Let stand around 5 minutes until thickened. In a bowl, whisk the salt, nutmeg, cloves, baking soda, xanthum gum, ginger, cinnamon, flours, and arrowroot starch. Using a mixer on low speed, add 1/3 of the flax seed mixture and 1/3 of the flour mixture until well blended. Repeat until all have been added and well blended. Scrape the batter into the baking pan and smooth the top. Bake around 45 minutes until a toothpick comes out clean when inserted in the center. Let cool. Makes 16 servings.

Tofu Chocolate Cake

Cake Ingredients:

1 1/4 cup whole wheat flour
1 1/2 tsp . baking soda
1 1/2 tsp . baking powder
1 tsp salt

1 cup melted sweetened chocolate chips
12 oz. firm silken tofu, cut in large chunks
3/4 cup cocoa powder
1 cup raw agave nectar
1 tablespoon vanilla

Chocolate Frosting Ingredients:

3/4 cup melted sweetened chocolate chips
1/4 cup agave nectar
1 tablespoon vegan margarine
1 tablespoon coconut oil
6 oz. firm silken tofu
1/2 cup cocoa powder
1/3 cup unsweetened coconut flakes

Preparation

You can use a 9 inch by 12 inch pan or 2 8-inch round cake pans. For frosting, melt chocolate chips. In a bowl, mix tofu, coconut oil, butter, agave nectar, and chocolate using a mixer until smooth. Add the cocoa powder slowly until you have a stiffness like frosting. Using a spoon stir in the coconut flakes. If it becomes to hard add a tablespoon of milk. Put in the refrigerator while you prepare the cake. Preheat the oven to 350 degrees Fahrenheit and grease the pans. Melt the chocolate chips as directed on package and set aside. In a bowl, combine salt, baking powder, baking soda, and flour, set aside. In a food processor add the tofu, melted chocolate, agave nectar, cocoa powder, and vanilla, blend until smooth. Pour this mixture into the dry ingredients and mix until you have a stiff batter. Spread into pans and bake for 20 minutes for the rectangular pan or 35 minutes for the round pans. Frost and enjoy. Makes 20 servings.

Pumpkin Cheesecake

Ingredients:

1 vegan pie crust
3 cups canned pumpkin puree 1 cup raw cashew pieces
1 1/4 cups unsweetened almond milk

4 tablespoons cornstarch
1/2 cup brown sugar
1 tsp cinnamon
1/2 tsp allspice
1/2 tsp nutmeg
1 tsp ginger
1/2 tsp salt
1 tablespoon lemon juice
2 tsp vanilla
3 tablespoons vegan butter

Preparation

Place the cashews in a bowl, cover with boiling water and set aside for 2 hours so the cashews become soft. Preheat oven to 325 degrees Fahrenheit. When the cashews are soft, drain, and mix well with the milk, cornstarch, and sugar until smooth. Add this mixture to a saucepan along with the vanilla, lemon juice, and spices. Using a whisk stir over medium low heat until it becomes thick. Add the pumpkin and the vegan butter. Blend with a whisk until smooth. Pour the filling into the pie shell. Smooth with a spatula. Bake for 1 hour. Turn off the oven but leave the pie inside the oven for another hour. Place in the refrigerator for 2 hours. Makes 12 servings.

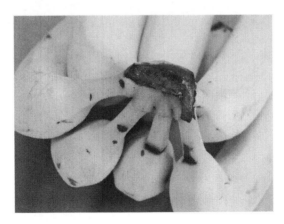

Açai Berry Banana Dessert

Ingredients

Samantha Michaels

4 single packages of amafruits pure unsweetened açaí fruit puree
24 oz frozen raspberries
1 cup unbleached cane sugar
½ cup powdered sugar
4 cups coconut cream
8 bananas

Preparation

Separate the coconut cream from the liquid in the cans of chilled coconut milk. Whip the cream with the powdered sugar using a mixer. Cover and chill in the refrigerator. Using the mixer on high speed, mix the acai berry puree, ½ of the frozen raspberries, and sugar, then chill. Allow the rest of the raspberries to thaw and drain. In dessert cups, add ¼ cup of the coconut cream, ½ cup of the acai raspberry pudding, 1 sliced banana, ¼ cup of coconut cream, 1 tablespoon thawed raspberries. Makes 8 servings.

Coconut Fruit Popsicles

Ingredients:

3 cups chopped sweet fruit
2/3 cup sugar
1/2 cup coconut milk

Preparation

You can use your favorite ripe fruit such as strawberries, blueberries, raspberries, or peaches. In a blender, puree all the ingredients. Fill the popsicle molds with the puree. Freeze for 3 hours. Can be stored in the freezer for one week. Makes 8 to 10 popsicles.

Coconut Fruit Tart

Ingredients

1 9-inch pre-baked pie crust
3 ½ cups coconut filling
2 ½ cups fresh fruit for topping

Coconut Filling Ingredients
3 1/2 cups coconut milk
3/4 cups water
3/4 cup sugar
1/4 tsp salt
1/2 cup cornstarch
1 1/2 tsp vanilla

Preparation

To make the filling, mix the water with the cornstarch, salt, and sugar. Set aside. In a pan, heat the coconut milk until steaming. Slowly whisk the cornstarch mixture into the milk. Continue cooking for around 15 minutes until the mixture is bubbly and thick, constantly stirring. Set aside and cool. Stir often to help release the steam. To make the fruit tart, spread the cooled filling in the pie crust. Cover with plastic wrap up against the filling so a fill will not form. Place in refrigerator for 4 hours. Arrange fruit on top before serving. Makes 12 servings.

Chocolate Raspberry Cookies

Ingredients:

1 cup ground toasted hazelnuts
1/4 cup white sugar
2 cups all-purpose flour
1/4 cup cocoa powder
1/4 tsp salt
1 cup vegan butter
1 cup white sugar
2 tablespoon tapioca flour and 2 tablespoons almond milk
1 tsp vanilla extract
1/2 cup semi-sweet chocolate chips
Powdered sugar
3/4 cup raspberry jam

Preparation

In a bowl, blend the salt, cocoa, flour, and tapioca flour, set aside. In another bowl, beat the sugar and butter until fluffy. Mix milk with the butter and sugar. Melt the chocolate chips and add to the butter mixture. Add the hazelnut mixture to the ingredients, blend well. Mix in the dry ingredients until well blended. Form the dough into 2 balls. Wrap and place in refrigerator for 1 hour. Preheat oven to 350 degrees Fahrenheit. Grease cookie sheets. Roll out the balls to ¼ inch thickness. Cut out the cookies. Bake cookies for 10 to 12 minutes. Dust the top cookies with powdered while spreading the bottom cookies with 1 tsp jam. Cover with the top cookies. Makes 20 cookies. Note: You can use any cookie cutters you desire to create these sandwiches cookies, just make sure the top cookie has a hole in the center so the jam can be seen.

Chocolate Fudge Brownies

Ingredients:

8 oz unsweetened vegan chocolate
1 cup vegan margarine
2 1/2 cups white sugar
2 1/2 tablespoon egg replacer
2/3 cup almond milk
1 tablespoon vanilla extract
2 1/2 cups flour
1/4 tsp salt
1 tsp baking soda
1 cup chopped walnuts

Frosting ingredients:

1 cup semisweet vegan chocolate chips
1/2 cup vegan margarine

Preparation

Preheat oven to 350 degrees Fahrenheit. Grease a 9 by 13 inch baking pan and dust with flour. In a saucepan, melt the butter and chocolate on low, set aside. Combine baking soda, salt, and flour, set aside. Whisk together the vanilla, milk, egg replacer, and sugar. Whisk the chocolate and butter and add to the milk mixture. Stir in the flour until blended. Add the walnuts and stir. Stir in the chocolate mixture. Spread the batter in the pan, bake 25 minutes.

Cool. To make the frosting, melt chocolate chips and let cool a bit. Cream the vegan butter, pour in the chocolate and mix until combined. Spread the frosting on the brownies. Makes 18 servings.

Lemon Cake

Lemon Cake Ingredients:

2/3 cup vegan butter
1 cup sugar
3 cups flour
3 Tablespoon cornstarch
2 1/2 tsp baking powder
1 tsp baking soda
1/4 tsp salt
1 1/2 cup non-dairy milk
Zest from 1 lemon
1/2 cup lemon juice

Lemon Frosting Ingredients:

1 cup vegan butter
1 lb powdered sugar
Zest from 2 lemons
1 tsp lemon extract
3 tablespoon lemon juice

Preparation

Preheat oven to 350 degrees Fahrenheit. Grease and dust a 9 by 12 or 2 9-inch cake pans. Mix the lemon juice and milk, set aside to curdle. Cream together the sugar and butter. Combine dry ingredients, then add to butter mixture along with the lemon zest and milk mixture. Mix until well blended. Spread the batter evenly in the pans and bake 35 to 45 minutes. Remove and cool. To make the frosting, blend the zest, sugar, and butter until smooth. Sift the sugar into the mixture using a strainer. Slowly beat in the lemon juice until the mixture has the consistency to spread easily. Place in the refrigerator until ready to use. Makes one cake.

Samantha Michaels

Baked Apples

Ingredients:

8 red apples
1 1/3 cup unbleached organic cane sugar
2 tsp cinnamon
6 tablespoon vegan
½ cup water

Preparation

Preheat oven to 350 degrees Fahrenheit. Wash the apples and cut a 1 ½ inch cone shape piece from around the stem of each apple. Use a spoon to get the rest of the core from the apples. Be sure not to break the other end of the apple. In a bowl, blend the butter, sugar, and cinnamon until you have a paste. Place 1/8 of the paste in the middle of each apple. Put the apples in a cake pan, add the water, cover, and bake 40 minutes until apples are tender. Makes 8 servings.

Citrus Pear Pomegranate Compote

Ingredients:

6 pears
4 cups of water
1/2 cup sugar
1 vanilla bean
1 tablespoon lemon juice
Juice from 1 lime
Juice and zest from 1 lemon
4 sectioned oranges
1/2 pomegranate
6 sprigs of fresh mint
Six serving bowls

Preparation

In a saucepan, combine the lemon zest, lemon juice, lime juice, vanilla bean, sugar, and water. Stir until sugar is completely dissolved. When the water begins to boil, lower heat and simmer. Prepare the pears, by peeling, quartering, and coring. Place them in the water. Simmer the pears for 5 minutes, remove and place in a bowl. Strain the syrup and pour over pears. Add the vanilla bean. Cover the bowl and chill in the refrigerator overnight. To serve, arrange the pears in each bowl, add the orange sections around the pears, sprinkle the pomegranate seeds over the pears, pour a little bit of the syrup over the pears. Garnish with the mint sprig. Makes 6 servings.

Peach Crumb Pie

Ingredients

Vegan pie crust
6 cups sliced peaches
1/2 cup water
1 1/2 tsp ground cinnamon
Crumb Topping:
1/2 cup unbleached all-purpose flour
1/2 cup granulated sweetener
2 tablespoon vegetable shortening

Preparation

Preheat oven to 400 degrees Fahrenheit. Grease a pie pan and set aside. Bake the pie crust for 10 minutes or until edges are lightly brown. To make the peach filling, place the peaches in a saucepan and add ¼ cup of water. Cover and cook until peaches are soft around 10 minutes. Add the cinnamon and stir gently. Remove from heat. In the water left in the pan, add the starch and stir. Add this mixture to the peaches. Pour the peaches into the pie crust. To make the topping, add all ingredients in a bowl and cut the shortening in until you have balls no larger than peas. Sprinkle the topping on the peaches. Bake for 10 minutes or until topping is brown. Makes 10 servings.

Samantha Michaels

MORE 70 BEST EVER RECIPES EBOOKS

REVEALED AT MY AUTHOR PAGE:-

CLICK HERE TO ACCESS THEM NOW

14594454R00037

Printed in Great Britain
by Amazon.co.uk, Ltd.,
Marston Gate.